WHY MACROBIOTICS IS MY FAVORITE BIG WORD

Emma Holister

Foreword by Michio Kushi

Note to the Reader: Those with health problems are advised to seek the guidance of a qualified medical or nutritional professional before implementing any of the recommendations in this book. It is essential that any reader who has any reason to suspect serious illness seek appropriate advice. Neither this nor any other book should be used as a substitute for qualified care or treatment.

Why Macrobiotics Is My Favorite Big Word
© 1998 by Emma Holister

For further information on mail-order sales, wholesale, or retail discounts, distribution, translations, and foreign rights, please contact the publisher: One Peaceful World Press, P.O. Box 10, Becket, MA 01223. U.S.A., telephone (413) 623-2322, fax (413) 623-6042.

First Edition: October 1998
ISBN 1-882984-33-1

To Mum and Dad
to Roy, Eleanor, and Simon Salisbury,
and to my lovely husband, José,
with gratitude and love

Foreword
By Michio Kushi

Emma Holister's new book is a wonderful way to help spread the good news about diet and health.

Over the last thirty years, thousands of people—men and women, boys and girls, young and old—have benefited from the macrobiotic way of life, including many with serious illness, including cancer.

The value of this dietary approach is now being recognized by society. The National Institutes of Health (NIH) has been researching macrobiotics and cancer. On its Internet site, the American Cancer Society states, "Today's most popular anticancer diet is probably macrobiotics," and refers to several medical studies showing the antitumor effects of macrobiotic-quality foods. The Smithsonian Institution is developing a collection on macrobiotics and alternative health care.

Major foods in the macrobiotic way of eating—including whole grains; beans and bean products such as miso, tofu, and tempeh; fresh vegetables; and sea vegetables—are increasingly served in schools, hospitals, and clinics as well as in homes, restaurants, and hotels.

I hope everyone—children and parents, teachers and grandparents—will be inspired by this volume. Like Lucy, the little girl in Emma's entertaining new book, "macrobiotics" is my favorite big word. After giving a balanced whole foods diet a chance, I hope it will be yours, too.

Hello. My name's Lucy, and I like big words. . . .

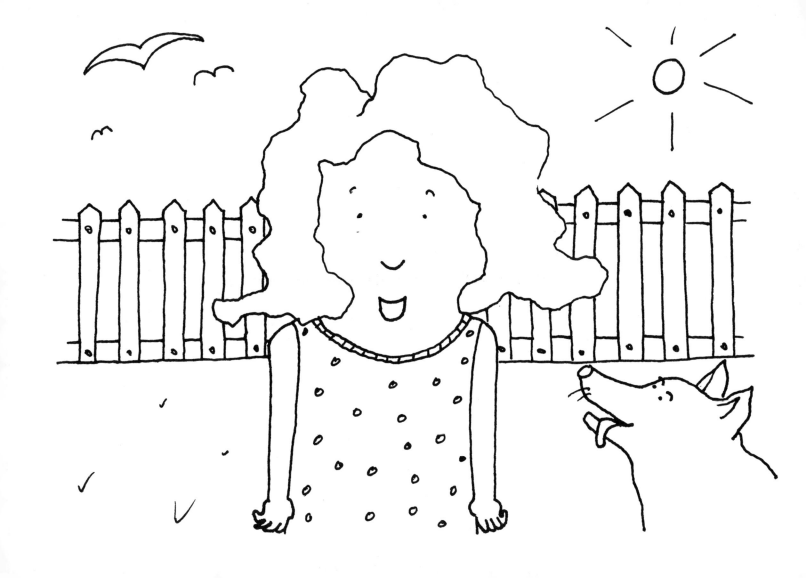

Sometimes people don't always understand what I'm saying. . . .

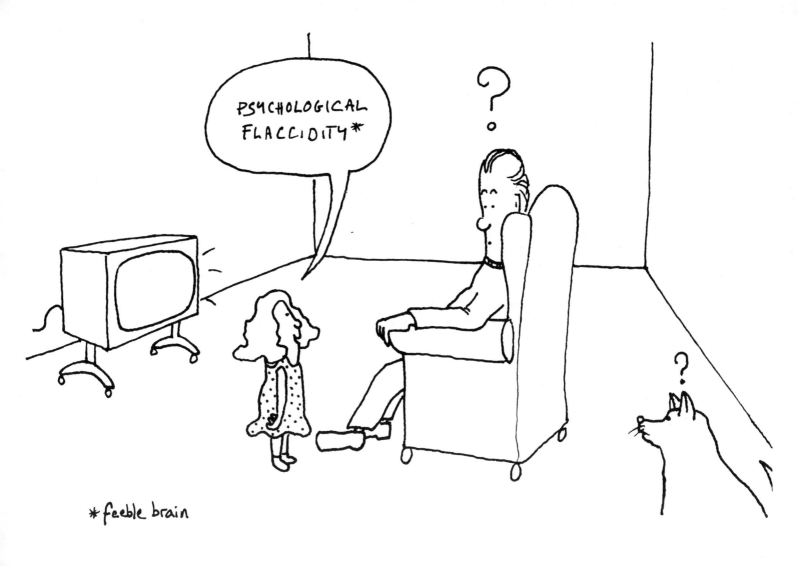

. . . So I'll try not to use too many.

One of my first ever favorite big words was "vegetarian." I'm a vegetarian. I don't eat meat because I like animals and I don't want to eat them,if you see what I mean.

My Mum and Dad used to eat a lot of meat, especially beef and pork. So from time to time, I would try to offer them a little friendly information. . . .

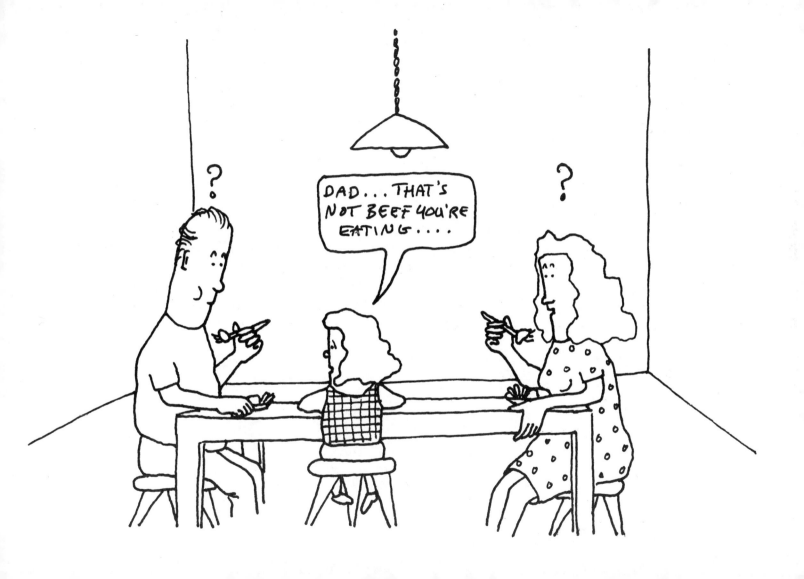

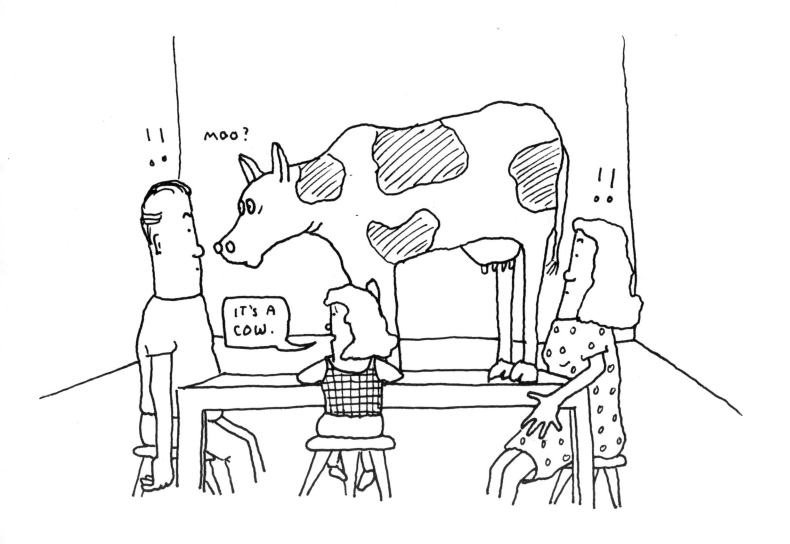

This is the story about how the word "macrobiotics" became my favorite big word.

My Mum wasn't feeling well so she went to the doctor's. He told her she had cervical cancer. A serious illness in the place in her tummy where babies come from.

We were all very worried.

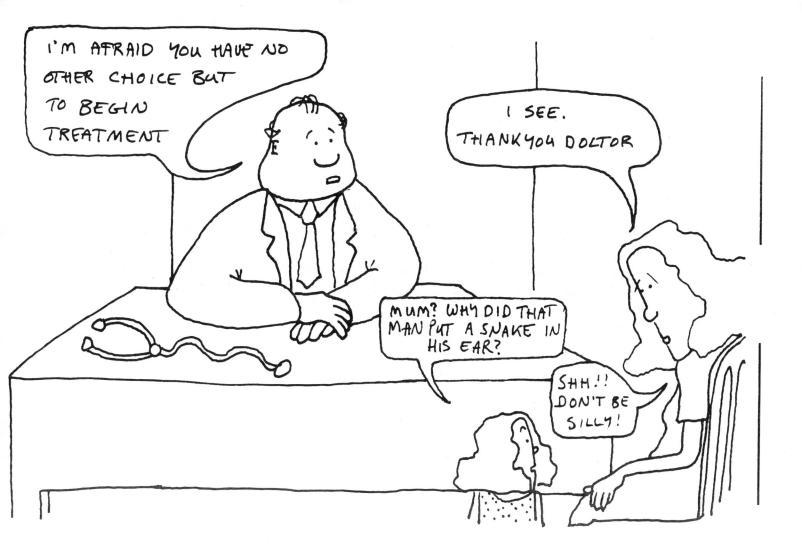

When Mum's friend, Brenda, found out she had cancer, she came round right away and gave Mum a book on the macrobiotic diet.

She said to keep listening to her doctor's advice and to go ahead with the treatment. But as her treatment wasn't for a while yet, to start the diet straight away. It could cure her.

Mum was very happy that she could do something to help herself. She decided to give it a try.

She gave up meat, sugary food and drinks, oily and fried food and dairy products, like cheese, milk, and eggs.

And she started cooking whole grains like brown rice and fresh organic vegetables and beans. . . .

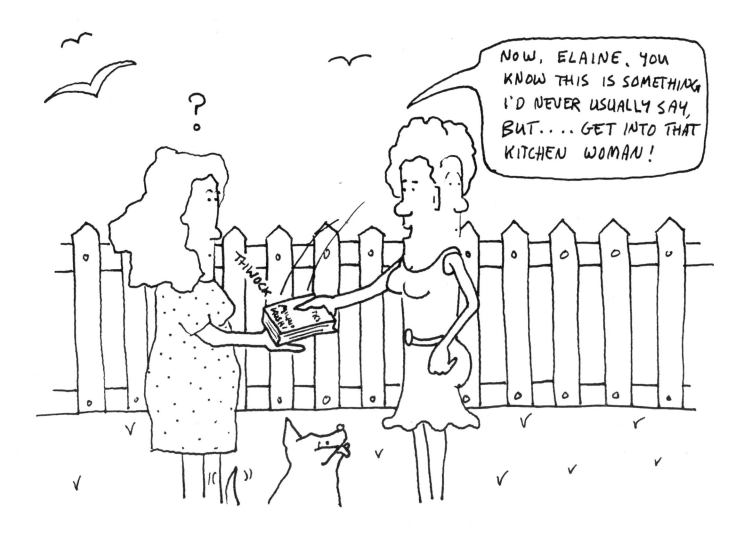

At first it didn't go too well. . . .

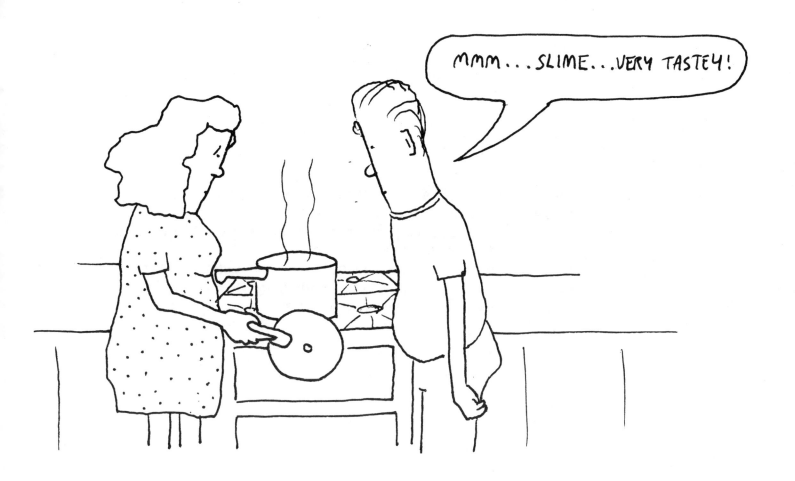

But Mum doesn't give up easily and she asked Brenda, who knew a lot about the macrobiotic diet, to come over and help her.

Dad made fun of Brenda and said she ate "macro-slime" and that Mum was going on the "macro-slime diet."

Mum said she would show him he was wrong and sent him out of the kitchen.

And before long, she proved that she was right. She began to make delicious, healthy meals. All she needed was patience, determination, and support from us.

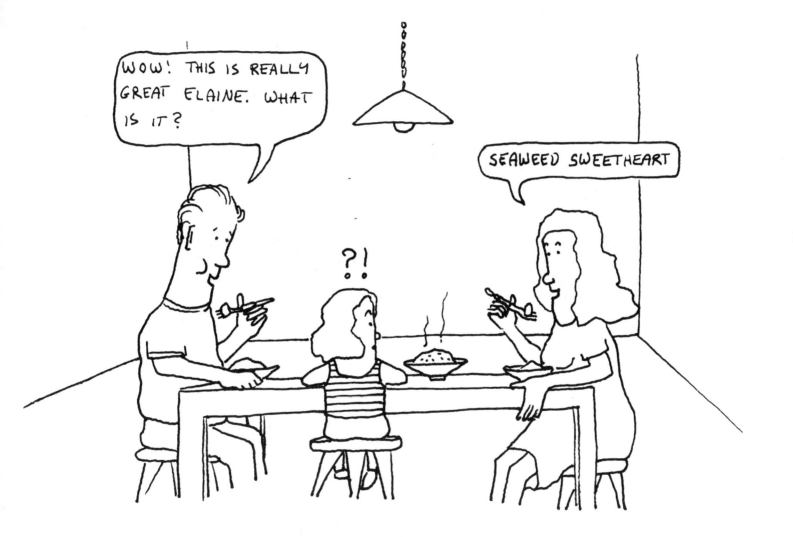

The person who wrote the book said it was also important to chew every mouthful at least 50 times, preferably 100 times. This is to make sure that when the food is swallowed, it is completely liquid. This improves digestion a lot and helps the body fight illness.

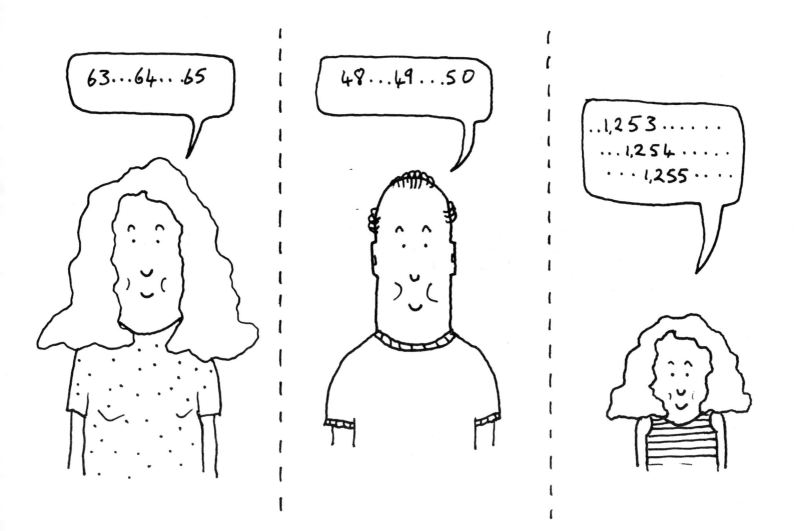

Going out and enjoying the beauty of nature was recommended and going out for walks everyday. Walking is an excellent form of exercise.

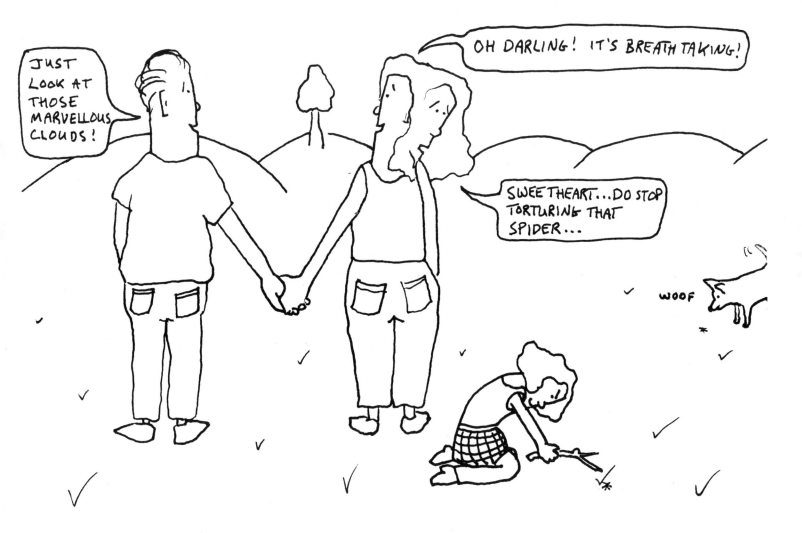

He also encouraged other forms of exercise.

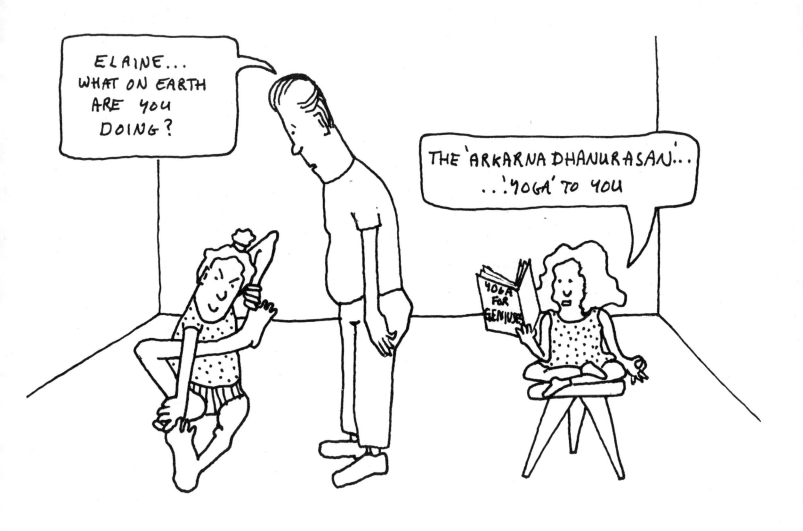

He said it was good to develop spiritually.

My Mum is a Buddhist, she believed in the mystic universal law of life. And my Dad is a Christian, he believes in God.

I like to see myself as an agnostic . . . I choose not to practice a religion . . . also It's a really good BIG WORD.

So while my Mum chants more . . .

. . . And my Dad prays more . . .

. . . I like to . . .

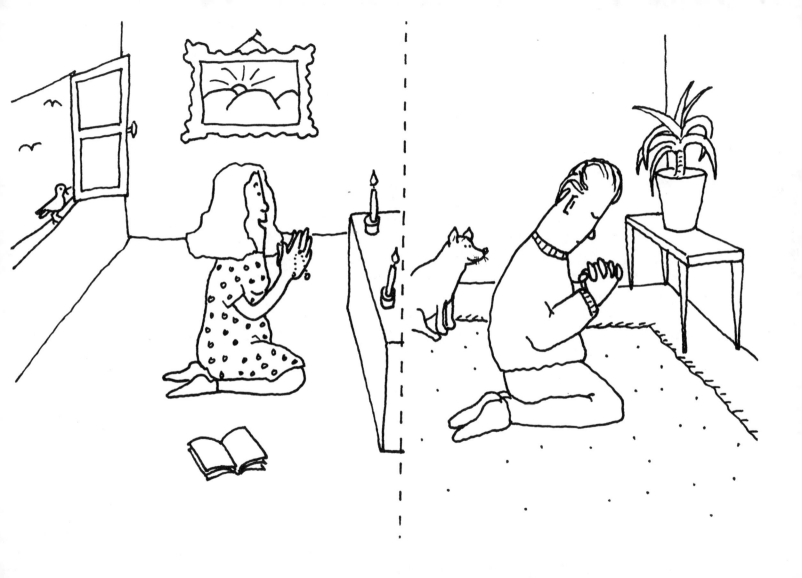

. . . develop my skills in levitation* . . .

* to lift yourself into the air through the power of your mind

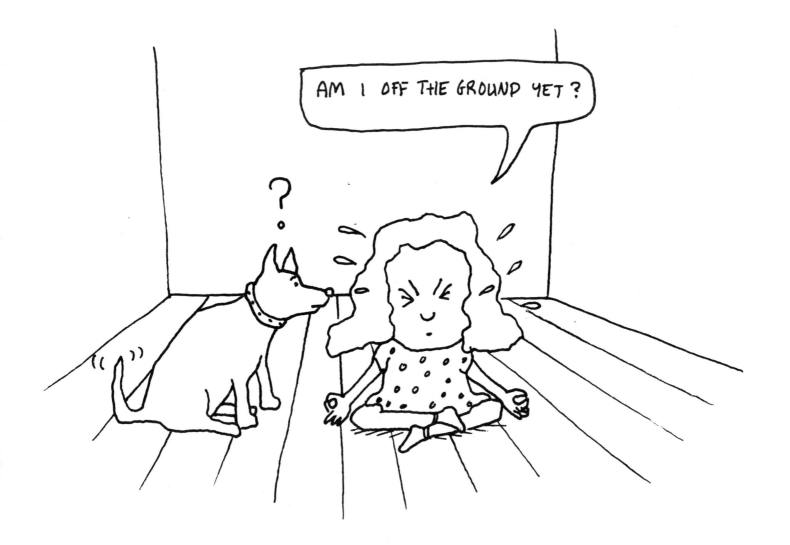

I didn't have much success with levitation, but something else happened which was really good.
Mum and Dad lost weight.

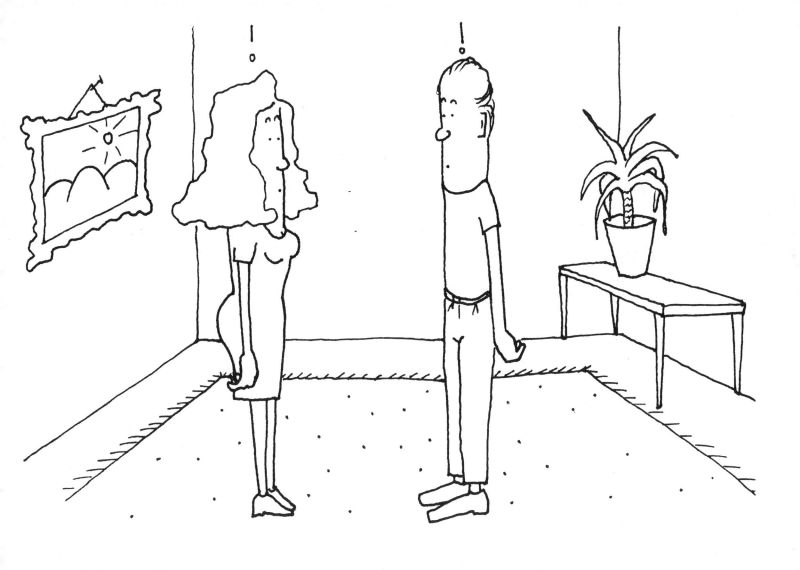

    They seemed to be falling in love with each other all over again, which was
great.
    Although I was a little concerned when they began to talk vegetable language
. . . .

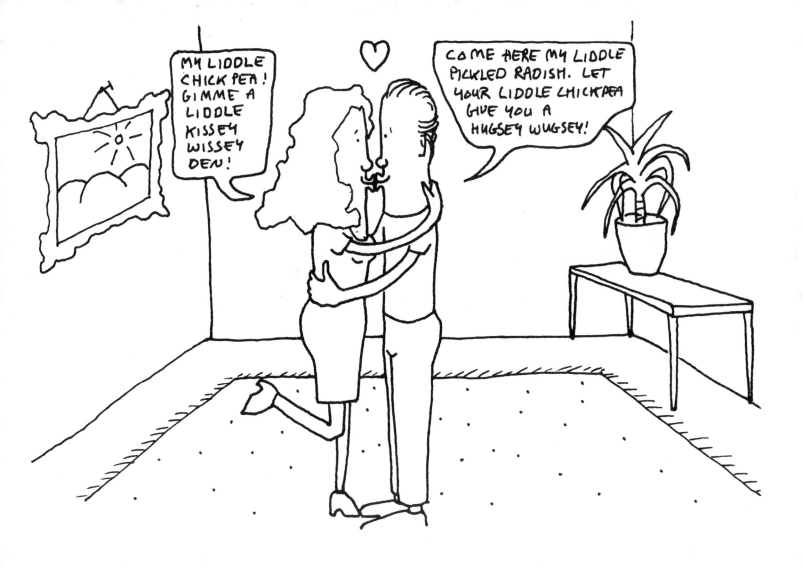

It wasn't just that they were slimmer and falling in love again . . . They had more energy in general. What's more, Mum stopped being so crabby and Dad stopped getting so stressed all the time.

In fact, I was amazed. They seemed so much younger altogether.

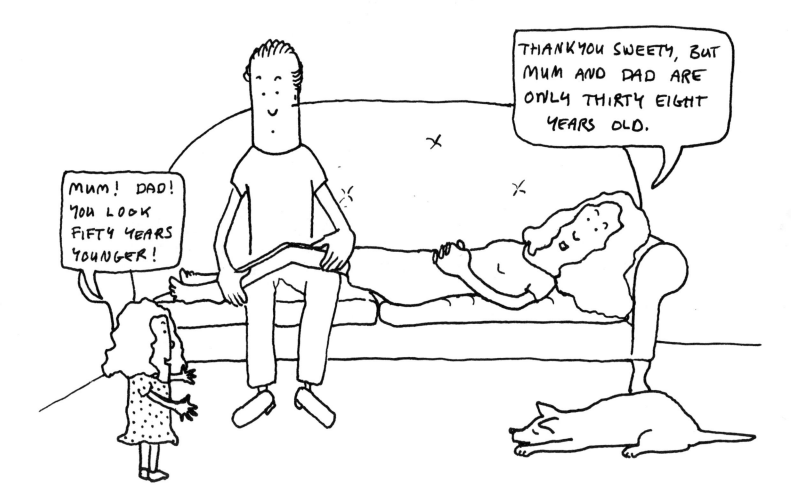

When Mum went back to the doctor's, he said that the cancer was "regressing." That means that it was shrinking. She seemed to be getting better.

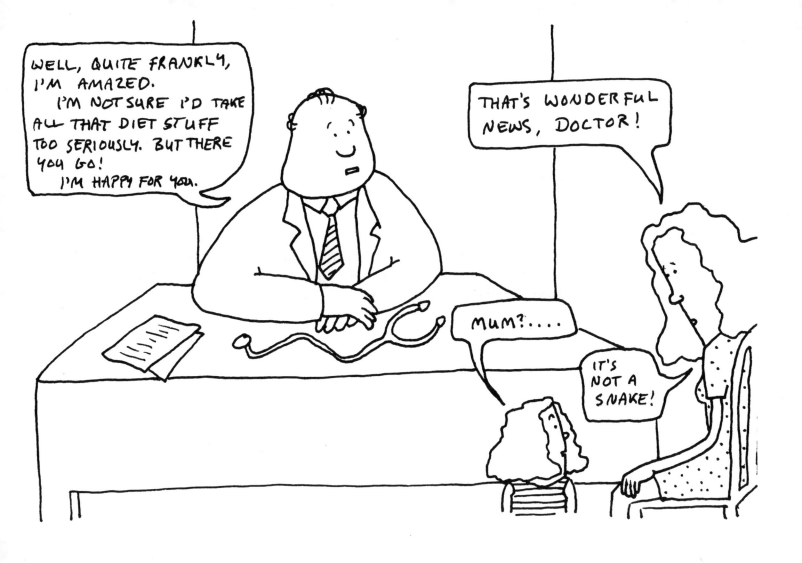

Now she knew for sure that the macrobiotic diet was working, she continued even harder, never forgetting to do all the other things that were recommended, like the home remedies, such as hip baths.

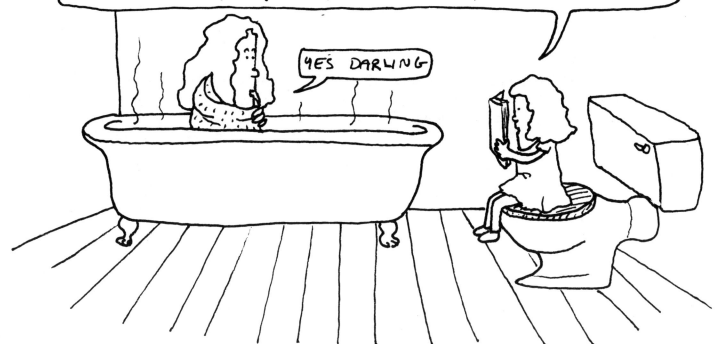

. . . And singing everyday. . . . Although I never understood why they said it is supposed to be relaxing.

They keep telling me that their favorite song is an old Motown classic . . .

Well, if that's what music from Motown sounds like, I never want to go there!

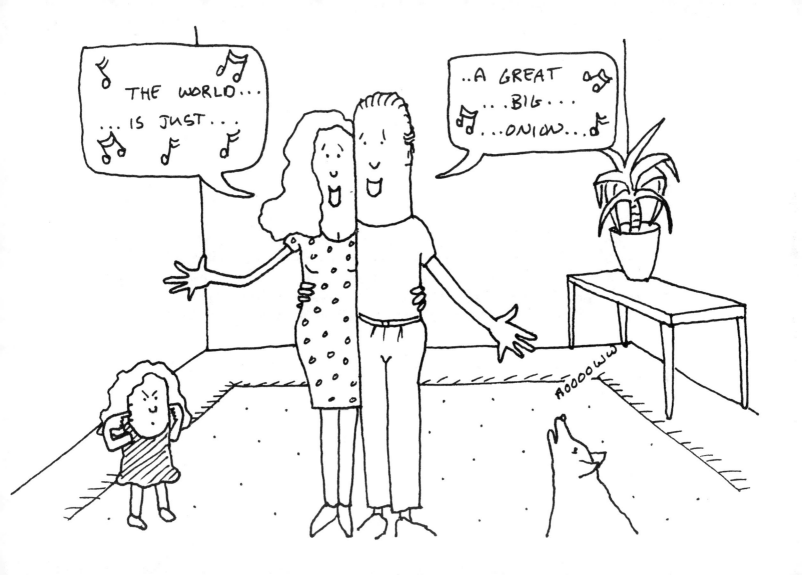

Apart from the horrible singing, a couple of good things happened . . . First of all, my excema went away when I stopped eating cheese and drinking milk.

Excema is when your skin goes dry, red, and itchy. Sometimes mine got so bad it would bleed. You can imagine how pleased I was that it went away.

And my Dad was delighted when his dandruff went away, too . . . So was Mum.

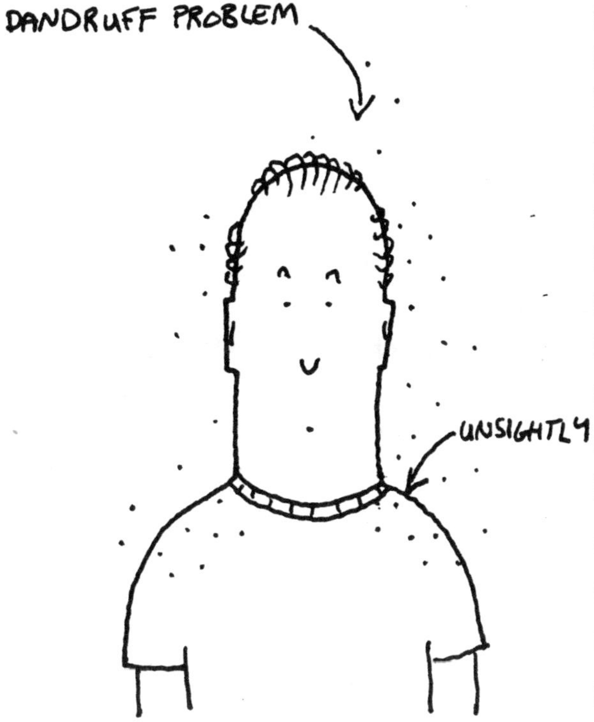
DANDRUFF PROBLEM
UNSIGHTLY

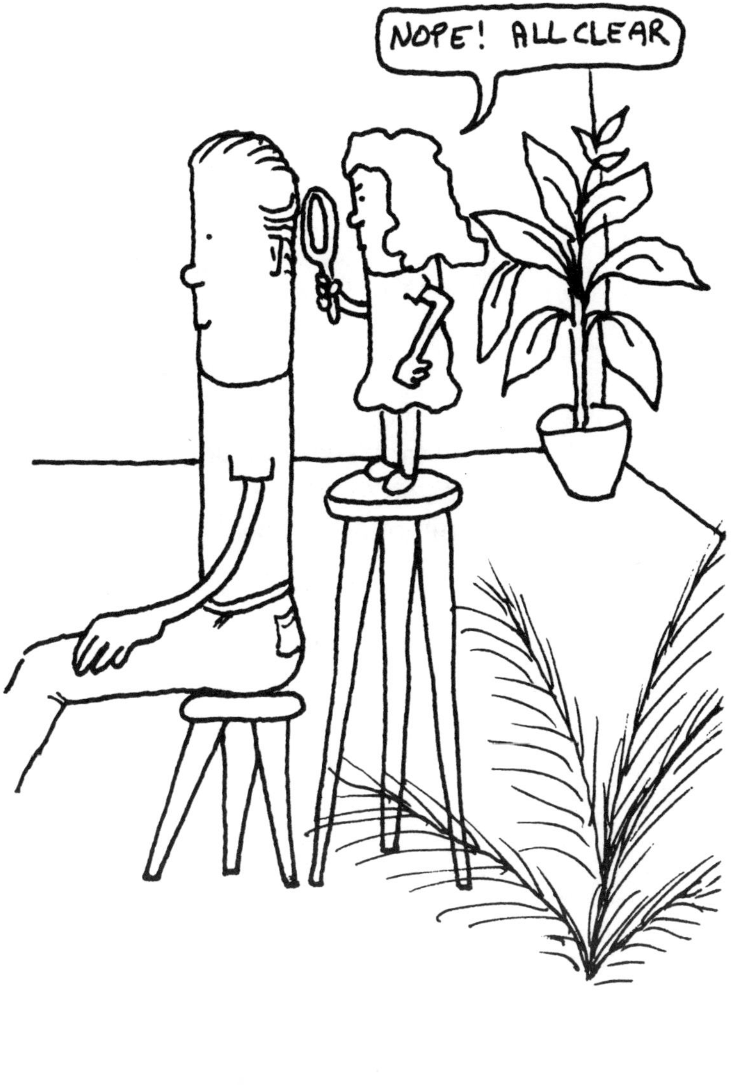
NOPE! ALL CLEAR

In fact, Dad was so pleased about his dandruff that he decided to take up cooking, too.
Although this did have rather a strange effect on Mum . . .

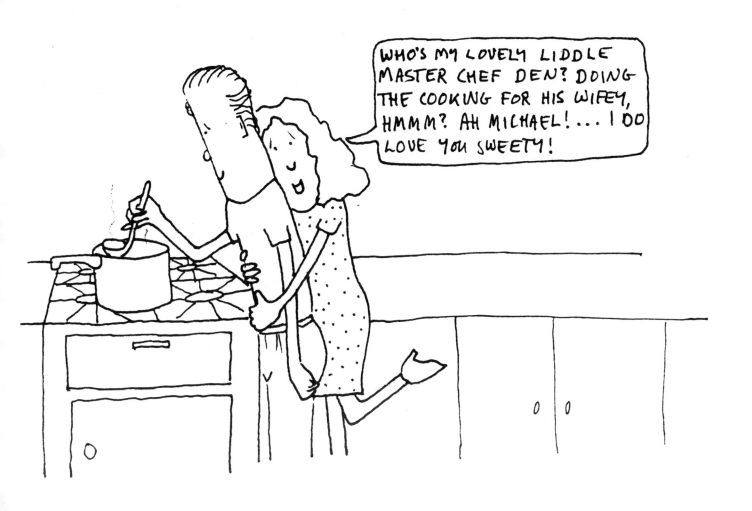

It wasn't just us that changed. The house changed, too. Dad had the house filled with plants, because they help clean the air and provide lots of oxygen for us to breathe.

Mum had read that doing daily breathing exercises was excellent for purifying the blood . . . she got quite carried away sometimes . . .

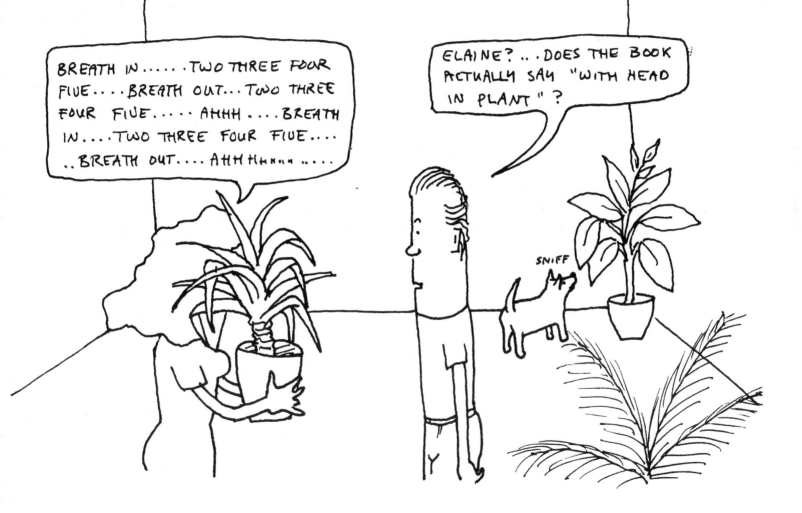

The next time we went to the doctor's he was off sick, but the nice lady who was replacing him gave us some wonderful news.

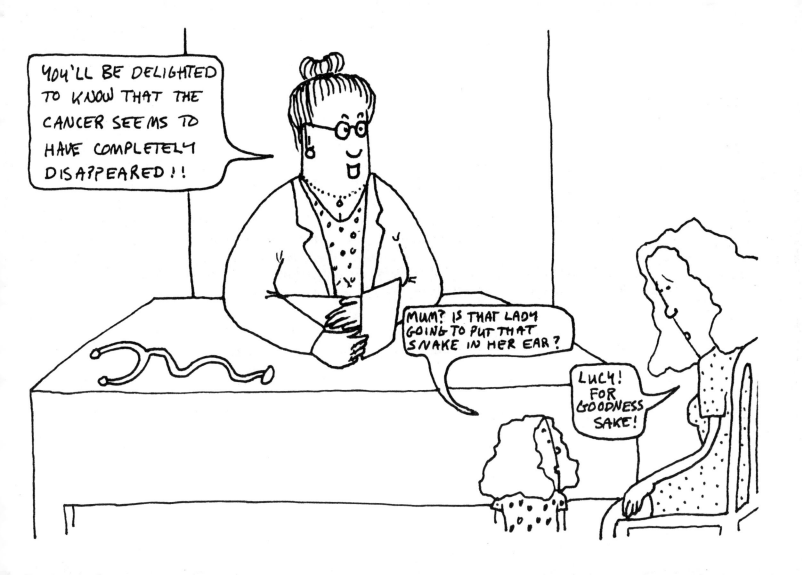

We were all very, very, very happy.

Mum even said that she was glad she had got cancer because thanks to her illness she was able to change lots of negative things in her life.

She sometimes said to me, "Just think, Lucy, if I had never got cancer, your Dad would never have got rid of his dandruff!" And then she laughs a lot . . . although I don't exactly know why.

I'm pleased because I learnt a new big word. That wasn't a snake after all in the doctor's office. It's what they use to hear people's hearts and lungs.

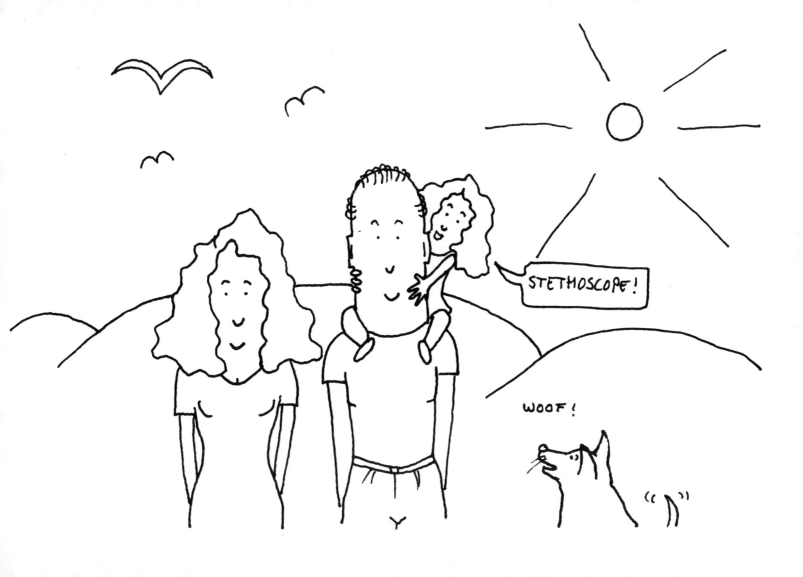

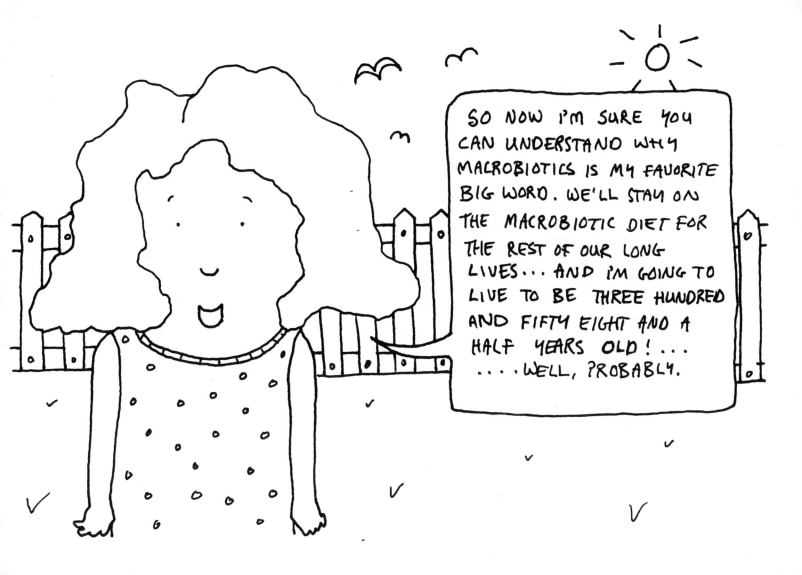

Afterword

By Emma Holister

Despite a few lingering bad food habits, I created this book because I have benefited immensely from the macrobiotic diet. In 1989 while living in Paris, doctors found I had a precancerous condition of the cervix and gave me an appointment for surgery a month later. Within two weeks of starting macrobiotics, my condition cleared up so dramatically that my physician told me the operation was no longer necessary.

Over the years, I had suffered from a long string of health problems, including bulemia, bronchitis, kidney infections, irritable bowel syndrome, seborrhea on the scalp, and yeast infections. All of these are now behind me. Today I enjoy radiant good health in Puerto Rico where I live with my husband.

Through my story and drawings, I wish to express my heartfelt gratitude to all those at the Kushi Institute and One Peaceful World who over the years have made it possible for thousands of people on the planet to radically improve their health and transform their lives.

I also hope this book will encourage and amuse people on the macrobiotic diet, above all, those just beginning and especially children. Keep it up! It really is worth it, you'll see.

A healthy body and a healthy mind are what we require to make this beautiful planet, genuinely, One Peaceful World.

Appendix
Some of My Favorite Recipes

Basic Brown Rice

I like to alternate my rice so that it is cooked with a different grain or bean every day (e.g., rice with millet one day, rice with barley the next, then rice with aduki beans or lentils, then plain rice, etc.)

1 cup organic short-grain brown rice
$1/2$ cup organic millet (or barley or aduki beans, etc.)
2 $1/4$ cups water (natural spring water preferably)
1-inch piece of kombu or 2 pinches of sea salt

Rinse and drain grains well before cooking. Put all the ingredients in a stainless steel pressure-cooker and bring to full pressure. Lower heat immediately to simmer and let cook for 50 minutes. Release pressure, remove lid, and let sit for several minutes.

Seitan with Shiitake Mushroom and Onion Gravy

1 medium sized onion, sliced thinly
4 shiitake mushrooms, sliced thinly (soak and rinse well beforehand)
1 clove garlic, crushed
1 cup of water
1 teaspoon of arrowroot dissolved in a little cold water (kuzu or flour may be
    substituted)
2 or 3 teaspoons shoyu
1 8-ounce package of seitan, broken into small chunks
1 teaspoon dark sesame oil

Fry onions and mushrooms gently in oil. When they begin to go brown, add garlic.
Cook for one more minute. Add water and shoyu and bring to a boil. Let simmer
for 1-2 minutes. Add dissolved arrowroot and stir constantly until it thickens. Add
seitan, cover, and simmer, stirring occasionally, until cooked through. Serve hot
with rice and steamed broccoli.

This sauce is also good on fried or steamed tofu or fried tempeh. Use ordinary
mushrooms if shiitakes are not available.

Chinese Cabbage

4 or 5 leaves of chinese cabbage, sliced into 3"x1" strips
1 teaspoon brown rice syrup
1 teaspoon brown rice vinegar
2 or 3 teaspoons shoyu
1 teaspoon arrowroot, dissolved in a little cold water

Heat oil, syrup, vinegar, and shoyu in a wok or skillet. Add cabbage and cook, stirring and covering occasionally until leaves begin to soften. (If liquid evaporates too quickly, add a little water.) Add arrowroot in its water and stir well until sauce thickens and sticks to cabbage. Serve hot.

Arame and Carrot Stir-Fry

2 cups cooked arame sea vegetable
1 carrot, sliced into matchsticks
1 onion, sliced thinly
2 teaspoons dark sesame oil
2 teaspoons brown rice vinegar

Fry carrot and onion in a wok or skillet with oil until cooked. Stir in cooked arame and vinegar. Stir-fry for a further minute. Serve immediately.

Barley Rice and Aduki Bean Salad

2 cups cooked brown rice with barley
1 teaspoon white miso
1/2 cup parsley, chopped very fine
1 carrot, chopped very fine
1 onion, sliced fine

Warm up the barley rice (see above basic rice recipe) in a pan and add a little white miso dissolved in a little water. Add other ingredients and toss lightly, adding brown rice vinegar to taste.

Roasted Sunflower or Pumpkin Seeds

1/2 cup seeds

Sort seeds for stones, etc. Place in a non-oiled pan and dry-roast, turning occasionally with a wooden spoon or paddle until they begin to go brown. You may also add a few drops of shoyu and stir in quickly. Toss seeds in a pan for a few more seconds to let shoyu dry onto them.

Resources

The One Peaceful World Society is an international information network and macrobiotic friendship society founded by Michio Kushi. Membership is $30 year for individuals ($40 outside of the U.S. and Canada) and $50 for families and benefits include the quarterly *One Peaceful World Journal*, a free book from One Peaceful World Press, and discounts on books and study materials. To join or for information, please contact: One Peaceful World, Box 10, Becket, MA 01223, (413) 623-2322, Fax (413) 623-6042.

The Kushi Institute is an educational center for macrobiotic and holistic studies. Several times a month, the Kushi Institute offers The Way to Health Program, a week-long seminar designed primarily for those with cancer or other serious illness and supporting family members or friends. The residential program includes daily hands-on cooking classes and theory classes. A dietary and way of life consultation, especially tailored to the individual's unique needs and conditions, is also available. For information, including seminar dates and costs, please contact: Kushi Institute, Box 7, Becket, MA 01223, (413) 623-5741, Fax (413) 623-8827.

Recommended Reading

Aveline Kushi's Complete Guide to Macrobiotic Cooking by Aveline Kushi with Alex Jack (Warner Books, $15.99). One of the best general cookbooks, including hundreds of recipes and Aveline's charming stories, drawings, and poems about growing up in Japan.

Basic Home Remedies by Michio Kushi (One Peaceful World Press, $6.95), guide to the 50 most common macrobiotic home cares, including ginger compress, lotus root plaster, and medicinal teas and drinks.

Basic Shiatsu by Michio Kushi with Edward Esko (One Peaceful World Press, $8.95), how to give a healthful, relaxing massage. Includes complete meridian charts.

Cancer-Free: 30 Who Overcame Cancer Naturally edited by Ann Fawcett (Japan Publications, $19.00) presents accounts by several dozen men and women who used macrobiotics to recover from cancer.

The Cancer-Prevention Diet by Michio Kushi with Alex Jack (St. Martin's Press, revised edition, $15.95) is the principal macrobiotic text on cancer and diet. Its nearly 500 pages include complete theoretical sections, individual chapters on the 20 most common types of cancer, including dietary recommendations, home cares, case histories, nutritional research, and menus and recipes.

Eat Your Veggies by Wendy Esko (One Peaceful World Press, $8.95), over 100 recipes for glorious greens, robust root vegetables, and succulent casseroles.

Healing Foods by Michio Kushi (One Peaceful World Press, $6.95), a handbook to over 50 nutritious foods that create health, balance energy, and prevent disease. Includes the most recent U.S. and Japanese food tables.

Raising Healthy Children by Michio and Aveline Kushi (Avery Publications, $14.95), a holistic approach to parenting and childcare, including home remedies and special foods for babies and children.

Rice Is Nice by Wendy Esko (One Peaceful World Press, $$8.95), 108 delicious and healthful brown rice recipes, including croquettes, rice balls, and sushi.

Soup du Jour by Wendy Esko (One Peaceful World Press, $8.95), over 100 delicious, hearty soups, broths, and stews.

Standard Macrobiotic Diet by Michio Kushi (One Peaceful World Press, $6.95), basic introduction to the macrobiotic way of eating, including guidelines for temperate, tropical, and cold regions, and a dozen recipes.

The Women's Health Guide edited by Gale Jack and Wendy Esko (One Peaceful World Press, $10.95), includes several case histories for breast cancer, uterine cancer, bulemia, endometriosis, and other conditions.

These and other other books are available from One Peaceful World Press, Box 10, Becket, MA 01223, (413) 623-2322, Fax (413) 623-6042. Please add $3.00 shipping per order.

About the Author

Emma Holister is an English-born artist and writer. She became macrobiotic after healing herself of a precancerous condition. Her work has been displayed in the U.K. and Puerto Rico where she presently lives with her husband. Her most recent project was an exhibition of oils on canvas to support the creation of safe houses for sufferers of domestic violence.

For further information, Emma may be contacted at Calle Lima P-326, Rolling Hills, Carolina, Puerto Rico 00987.